SJOGREN'S SYNDROME DIET COOKBOOK

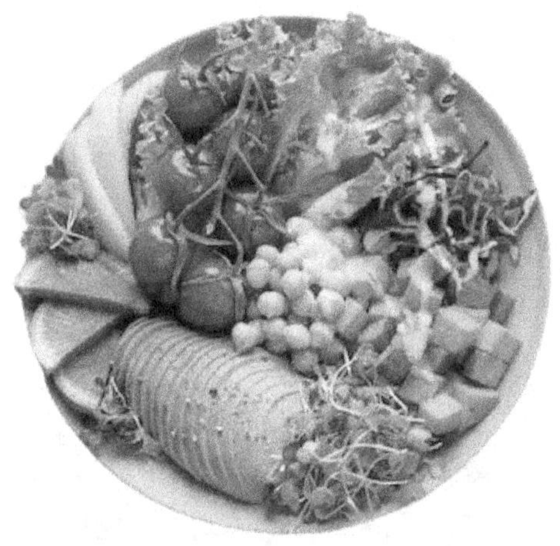

BY

DR. VICKIE STOCK

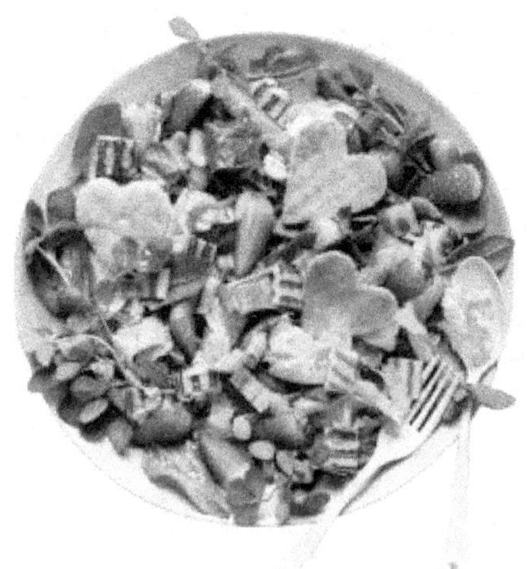

TABLE OF CONTENT

CHAPTER ONE

Introduction to Sjögren's Syndrome:

Sjögren's syndrome, named after the Swedish ophthalmologist Henrik Sjögren who first described it in 1933, is a chronic autoimmune disorder that primarily affects the exocrine glands, leading to symptoms of dryness in various parts of the body.

This complex and often underdiagnosed condition can have a profound impact on a person's quality of life, affecting not only their physical well-being but also their emotional and social dimensions.

At its core, Sjögren's syndrome is characterized by the immune system's misguided attack on the body's moisture-producing glands, such as the salivary and lacrimal glands.

This autoimmune response results in a reduction of saliva and tears, causing dryness in the mouth and eyes, which are hallmark symptoms of the syndrome. However, Sjögren's can extend beyond these primary symptoms, affecting other organs and systems throughout the body.

One of the distinctive features of Sjögren's syndrome is its classification into two main types: primary and secondary. Primary Sjögren's occurs when the syndrome exists on its own, without any other underlying autoimmune condition. On the other hand, secondary Sjögren's syndrome is diagnosed when it coexists with another autoimmune disorder, often rheumatoid arthritis or lupus.

The symptoms of Sjögren's syndrome can be diverse and vary from person to person. Beyond the hallmark dryness of the mouth and eyes, individuals with Sjögren's may experience fatigue, joint pain, and various complications affecting internal organs.

The syndrome's systemic nature can lead to complications ranging from dental issues due to reduced saliva, to more serious conditions such as lung and kidney involvement.

The diagnostic journey for Sjögren's syndrome can be challenging, as its symptoms overlap with those of other autoimmune disorders. Healthcare professionals often rely on a combination of clinical evaluations, blood tests, and imaging studies to reach an accurate diagnosis.

Early detection is crucial to managing the symptoms and preventing potential complications.

Living with Sjögren's syndrome requires a multidisciplinary approach to address the diverse range of symptoms and complications.

Treatment plans typically focus on alleviating dryness through artificial tears, saliva substitutes, and medications to modulate the immune response. Additionally, managing associated symptoms like joint pain and fatigue is integral to improving overall quality of life for those affected.

In recent years, research into Sjögren's syndrome has expanded, shedding light on the underlying mechanisms and paving the way for potential targeted therapies.

Clinical trials and advancements in understanding the genetic and environmental factors contributing to the development of Sjögren's offer hope for more effective treatments in the future.

Despite the challenges posed by Sjögren's syndrome, individuals with the condition often find support through patient advocacy groups, online communities, and healthcare professionals specializing in autoimmune disorders. The journey with Sjögren's is a complex one, but with ongoing research and a comprehensive approach to care, there is hope for improved management and, ultimately, a better quality of life for those affected by this intricate autoimmune disorder.

What is Sjogren's syndrome

Sjögren's syndrome is a chronic autoimmune disorder characterized by the immune system's attack on moisture-producing glands, leading to widespread dryness, particularly in the eyes and mouth.

Named after the Swedish physician Henrik Sjögren who first identified it, this condition affects both women and men, although it is more prevalent in females. The hallmark symptoms of Sjögren's include dry eyes, dry mouth, and difficulty swallowing, which can significantly impact an individual's daily life and overall well-being.

In addition to the primary symptoms, Sjögren's syndrome can manifest systemically, affecting various organs and systems throughout the body. Individuals with Sjögren's may experience fatigue, joint pain, and complications involving the respiratory, gastrointestinal, and genitourinary systems.

The syndrome can occur as a standalone condition, known as primary Sjögren's, or in conjunction with other autoimmune diseases, referred to as secondary Sjögren's.

Diagnosing Sjögren's syndrome can be complex, often involving a combination of clinical assessments, blood tests measuring specific antibodies, and imaging studies to evaluate gland function.

While there is currently no cure for Sjögren's, treatment aims to alleviate symptoms and may include artificial tears, saliva substitutes, and medications to modulate the immune response.

Living with Sjögren's syndrome necessitates a comprehensive and individualized approach to managing symptoms and improving overall quality of life, often involving a collaborative effort between patients and healthcare professionals.

Ongoing research into the underlying mechanisms of Sjögren's holds promise for more targeted and effective therapies in the future.

Sjogren's Syndrome Symptoms and Diagnosis

Symptoms of Sjögren's Syndrome:

Sjögren's syndrome manifests with a diverse range of symptoms that can significantly impact various organ systems.

The hallmark features of the condition primarily revolve around dryness, affecting the eyes, mouth, and other mucous membranes.

Dry eyes can lead to irritation, a gritty sensation, and, in severe cases, damage to the cornea. Similarly, dry mouth, or xerostomia, can result in difficulty swallowing, speaking, and an increased susceptibility to dental issues such as cavities.

Beyond dryness, individuals with Sjögren's often experience fatigue, which can be debilitating and affect daily functioning. Joint pain, swelling, and stiffness are common, resembling symptoms seen in rheumatoid arthritis. The syndrome's systemic nature may lead to complications involving the respiratory and gastrointestinal systems, causing chronic cough, difficulty breathing, and digestive problems.

Moreover, Sjögren's syndrome can impact vital organs such as the kidneys, liver, and lungs. In some cases, neurologic manifestations like peripheral neuropathy may occur. Additionally, individuals may face challenges with concentration and memory, a condition often referred to as "brain fog."

Given the wide array of symptoms, the impact on quality of life can be substantial. Emotional well-being may be affected as individuals navigate the chronic nature of the disease and its associated challenges. Recognizing and addressing these symptoms comprehensively is crucial for managing Sjögren's syndrome effectively.

Diagnosis of Sjögren's Syndrome:

Diagnosing Sjögren's syndrome is a complex process that requires a combination of clinical evaluation, laboratory tests, and sometimes imaging studies. Since its symptoms overlap with those of other autoimmune disorders, a thorough medical history and physical examination are essential components of the diagnostic process.

Blood tests play a crucial role in identifying specific antibodies associated with Sjögren's, such as anti-SSA (Ro) and anti-SSB (La).

Elevated levels of these antibodies can provide important diagnostic clues. Additionally, tests measuring markers of inflammation, such as erythrocyte sedimentation rate (ESR) and C-reactive protein (CRP), may be conducted.

Imaging studies, such as salivary gland scintigraphy and ultrasound, can help assess the function and structure of the glands, aiding in the diagnosis. In some cases, a lip biopsy may be recommended to examine salivary gland tissue for characteristic inflammatory changes.

The diagnostic process requires a collaborative effort between patients and healthcare professionals, often involving rheumatologists, ophthalmologists, and oral health specialists.

Given the complexity of Sjögren's syndrome, early and accurate diagnosis is crucial for implementing effective management strategies and improving the overall quality of life for individuals living with this autoimmune disorder.

Sjogren's Syndrome Causes and Risk factor

Causes of Sjögren's Syndrome:

The exact cause of Sjögren's syndrome remains elusive, but it is widely recognized as an autoimmune disorder. In autoimmune conditions, the immune system, which is designed to protect the body from harmful invaders like bacteria and viruses, mistakenly attacks its own tissues.

In the case of Sjögren's, the immune system targets the moisture-producing glands, particularly the salivary and lacrimal glands, responsible for producing saliva and tears.

Genetic factors play a role in predisposing individuals to autoimmune diseases, and there is evidence to suggest a familial component in Sjögren's syndrome.

Certain genetic markers may increase susceptibility, but a specific genetic mutation directly causing the syndrome has not been identified. Environmental factors, such as viral infections, are also believed to trigger the onset of Sjögren's in genetically predisposed individuals. Epstein-Barr virus, in particular, has been linked to an increased risk.

Hormonal factors, particularly the role of estrogen, have been explored as well, given the higher prevalence of Sjögren's syndrome in women. Estrogen is thought to influence the immune system, and changes in hormone levels may contribute to the development or exacerbation of the syndrome. However, the interplay between genetics, environment, and hormones in Sjögren's remains an area of ongoing research.

Sjögren's Syndrome Risk Factors:

Sjögren's syndrome is a complex autoimmune disorder with a multifactorial etiology, and while the exact cause remains unclear, several risk factors have been identified that may contribute to the development of the condition.

Gender and Age:

Sjögren's syndrome predominantly affects women, with a female-to-male ratio of approximately 9:1. Hormonal factors, including estrogen fluctuations, are believed to play a role in the increased susceptibility of women. The majority of individuals are diagnosed between the ages of 40 and 60, although the syndrome can occur at any age.

Genetic Factors:

There is evidence to suggest a genetic predisposition to Sjögren's syndrome. Individuals with a family history of autoimmune disorders, such as rheumatoid arthritis or lupus, may have an elevated risk of developing Sjögren's. Certain genetic markers, particularly those associated with immune system regulation, have been identified in individuals with the syndrome.

Other Autoimmune Conditions:

Sjögren's syndrome often coexists with other autoimmune disorders, such as rheumatoid arthritis, systemic lupus erythematosus, and scleroderma. Having one autoimmune condition may increase the likelihood of developing additional autoimmune disorders, including Sjögren's.

Viral Infections:

Certain viral infections, such as Epstein-Barr virus (EBV), have been implicated as potential triggers for Sjögren's syndrome. The immune response to these infections may set the stage for the development of autoimmune conditions, including the attack on moisture-producing glands seen in Sjögren's.

Environmental Factors:

Environmental factors, including exposure to certain toxins or infections, may contribute to the development of Sjögren's syndrome. While the specific triggers remain elusive, environmental factors are believed to interact with genetic predisposition, potentially initiating or exacerbating the autoimmune response.

Hormonal Factors:

Hormonal fluctuations, particularly those related to estrogen levels, may influence the development and progression of Sjögren's syndrome. Women experiencing hormonal changes due to pregnancy, menopause, or oral contraceptive use may be at an increased risk.

Understanding these risk factors is essential for identifying individuals who may be more susceptible to Sjögren's syndrome. While these factors contribute to the overall risk, it's important to note that many individuals diagnosed with Sjögren's may not have any identifiable risk factors, highlighting the complexity of the interplay between genetic, hormonal, and environmental elements in the development of this autoimmune condition.

CHAPTER TWO

Sjögren's Syndrome Treatment:

Managing Sjögren's syndrome is a dynamic and multifaceted process that aims to alleviate symptoms, prevent complications, and improve overall quality of life for individuals affected by this autoimmune disorder.

While there is no cure for Sjögren's, a combination of pharmacological interventions, lifestyle adjustments, and supportive therapies form the foundation of treatment.

Symptomatic Relief:

Addressing the hallmark symptoms of dry eyes and dry mouth is paramount in Sjögren's treatment. Artificial tears, lubricating eye drops, and prescription medications that stimulate saliva production or act as saliva substitutes are commonly used to alleviate dryness and enhance comfort.

Immunomodulatory Medications:

For individuals with more severe symptoms or systemic manifestations of Sjögren's, immunomodulatory medications may be prescribed.

Corticosteroids and disease-modifying antirheumatic drugs (DMARDs) such as hydroxychloroquine can help modulate the immune response and reduce inflammation, thereby managing joint pain and other systemic complications.

Moisture Retention Strategies:

Beyond medication, incorporating moisture retention strategies is crucial. This includes maintaining adequate hydration, using humidifiers in living spaces to combat dry air, and avoiding environmental factors that exacerbate dryness, such as smoke and wind.

Dental Care:

Regular dental check-ups are essential for individuals with Sjögren's to address the increased risk of dental decay and infections due to reduced saliva production.

Good oral hygiene practices, fluoride treatments, and preventive measures can help manage dental complications associated with the syndrome.

Systemic Complications Management:

Individuals with Sjögren's may require specialized care for systemic complications that affect organs such as the lungs, kidneys, and liver. Collaborative efforts between rheumatologists and specialists in these areas are crucial to monitor and manage these complications effectively.

Physical and Occupational Therapy:

Physical and occupational therapy may be recommended to manage joint pain and stiffness, improve mobility, and enhance overall functional ability. These therapies play a vital role in maintaining physical well-being and preventing long-term disability.

Patient Education and Support:

Patient education is an integral aspect of Sjögren's management. Providing individuals with information about the condition, self-care strategies, and coping mechanisms empowers them to actively participate in their treatment plan.

Support groups and counseling can also play a crucial role in addressing the emotional and psychological impact of living with a chronic autoimmune disorder.

Tailoring the treatment plan to individual needs is key, as Sjögren's syndrome can vary widely among affected individuals. Regular follow-up appointments with healthcare providers allow for ongoing assessment and adjustments to the treatment strategy based on the progression of symptoms and potential complications. The goal is to optimize the balance between controlling the autoimmune response and preserving the individual's quality of life.

Complications of Sjögren's Syndrome:

Sjögren's syndrome, beyond its hallmark symptoms of dry eyes and dry mouth, can lead to various complications affecting multiple organ systems. Understanding and addressing these complications is crucial for comprehensive management and improved outcomes for individuals living with Sjögren's.

Dental Complications:

Reduced saliva production increases the risk of dental complications such as cavities, gum disease, and oral infections. Regular dental check-ups, good oral hygiene practices, and preventive measures are essential to minimize the impact on oral health.

Pulmonary Complications:

Sjögren's syndrome can affect the lungs, leading to conditions such as interstitial lung disease. Individuals may experience chronic cough, shortness of breath, and other respiratory symptoms. Pulmonary function tests and imaging studies are used to assess and monitor lung involvement.

Renal Complications:

In some cases, Sjögren's can lead to kidney involvement, resulting in conditions like interstitial nephritis or renal tubular acidosis. Monitoring kidney function through regular blood and urine tests is important to detect and manage renal complications.

Neurological Complications:

Peripheral neuropathy, a condition affecting the nerves outside the brain and spinal cord, can occur in individuals with Sjögren's syndrome. This may manifest as tingling, numbness, or weakness in the extremities.

Neurological assessments and diagnostic studies are employed to identify and manage these complications.

Lymphoma Risk:

Individuals with Sjögren's syndrome have an increased risk of developing lymphoma, a type of blood cancer. Regular monitoring and surveillance for signs of lymphoma, such as swollen lymph nodes, are crucial for early detection and intervention.

Gastrointestinal Complications:

Sjögren's can affect the gastrointestinal tract, leading to issues such as esophageal reflux and difficulty swallowing. Dietary modifications, medications, and lifestyle adjustments may be recommended to manage these complications.

Emotional and Psychological Impact:

Living with a chronic autoimmune disorder can take a toll on an individual's emotional and psychological well-being.

The challenges of managing symptoms, potential complications, and the impact on daily life may contribute to anxiety and depression. Supportive therapies, counseling, and patient education play a crucial role in addressing the emotional aspect of Sjögren's.

Managing complications often requires a multidisciplinary approach, involving rheumatologists, pulmonologists, nephrologists, and other specialists depending on the affected organ systems.

Regular follow-up appointments and ongoing assessments are essential to detect and address complications early, optimizing the overall care and quality of life for individuals with Sjögren's syndrome.

Nutrition Strategies to Improve Symptoms of Sjögren's Syndrome:

Sjögren's syndrome, characterized by dryness in the eyes and mouth along with a range of systemic symptoms, can significantly impact an individual's quality of life.

While there is no cure for Sjögren's, adopting a well-balanced and supportive nutritional approach can help manage symptoms and enhance overall well-being.

Hydration is Key:

Given the primary symptom of dryness, adequate hydration is crucial. Sipping water throughout the day helps combat the effects of reduced saliva and minimizes the risk of dehydration. Additionally, including hydrating foods like watermelon, cucumber, and celery can contribute to overall fluid intake.

Omega-3 Fatty Acids:

Foods rich in omega-3 fatty acids, such as fatty fish (salmon, mackerel, and sardines), flaxseeds, and walnuts, possess anti-inflammatory properties. These can be beneficial for individuals with Sjögren's, as inflammation is a key component of autoimmune disorders.

Anti-Inflammatory Diet:

Emphasizing an anti-inflammatory diet may help alleviate joint pain and reduce inflammation associated with Sjögren's. This involves incorporating fruits, vegetables, whole grains, and lean proteins while minimizing processed foods, saturated fats, and sugars.

Vitamin D and Calcium:

Sjögren's patients may be at an increased risk of vitamin D deficiency, which can impact bone health. Adequate levels of vitamin D, obtained through sunlight exposure and supplementation if necessary, along with calcium-rich foods like dairy products, leafy greens, and fortified plant-based alternatives, can support bone health.

Soft and Moist Foods:

Dry mouth can make chewing and swallowing challenging. Opting for soft and moist foods, such as soups, stews, and smoothies, can make meals more palatable and facilitate easier swallowing.

Sugar-Free Gum and Candy:

Sugar-free gum or candy can stimulate saliva production, providing relief for dry mouth. However, it's important to choose products without artificial sweeteners, as they can sometimes exacerbate symptoms for some individuals.

Probiotics:

Probiotics, found in yogurt, kefir, and fermented foods, can support gut health and potentially modulate the immune system. Maintaining a healthy balance of gut bacteria may positively influence the overall immune response in autoimmune conditions.

Limit Caffeine and Alcohol:

Both caffeine and alcohol can contribute to dehydration, exacerbating dryness symptoms. Limiting intake and ensuring adequate water consumption is crucial for managing these aspects of Sjögren's.

Moderate Salt Intake:

Managing salt intake is important for individuals with Sjögren's, especially those dealing with kidney involvement. A balanced approach to salt can help control blood pressure and reduce the risk of associated complications.

Consultation with a Registered Dietitian:

Given the complexity of managing Sjögren's symptoms through nutrition, individuals may benefit from consulting with a registered dietitian.

A professional can tailor dietary recommendations to specific needs, considering individual preferences, nutritional deficiencies, and potential interactions with medications.

It's essential for individuals with Sjögren's syndrome to work collaboratively with healthcare professionals, including rheumatologists and registered dietitians, to create a comprehensive management plan that addresses both medical and nutritional aspects.

While nutrition alone cannot cure Sjögren's, adopting a thoughtful and supportive dietary approach can contribute to an improved quality of life for those navigating the challenges of this autoimmune disorder.

Foods to Include in a Sjögren's Syndrome Diet:

Omega-3 Rich Foods:

Fatty fish such as salmon, mackerel, and sardines, as well as flaxseeds and walnuts, are abundant in omega-3 fatty acids. These have anti-inflammatory properties that may help mitigate symptoms associated with Sjögren's syndrome.

Hydrating Fruits and Vegetables:

Water-rich fruits and vegetables like watermelon, cucumber, celery, oranges, and berries can contribute to overall hydration and alleviate dry mouth symptoms.

Soft and Moist Foods:

Opt for soft and moist foods like soups, stews, and casseroles to make chewing and swallowing more comfortable, especially if dry mouth is a prevalent symptom.

Probiotic-Rich Foods:

Yogurt, kefir, sauerkraut, and other fermented foods contain probiotics that can support gut health. A balanced gut microbiome may positively influence the immune system.

Calcium and Vitamin D Sources:

Incorporate dairy products, fortified plant-based alternatives, leafy greens, and fish with edible bones to ensure adequate calcium intake. Sun exposure and vitamin D supplements can also help support bone health.

Sugar-Free Gum or Candy:

Sugar-free gum or candy can stimulate saliva production, providing relief for dry mouth. Choose products without artificial sweeteners, as these can sometimes worsen symptoms for some individuals.

Lean Proteins:

Include lean proteins like poultry, fish, tofu, and legumes in your diet. Protein is essential for muscle health and overall well-being.

Whole Grains:

Opt for whole grains like brown rice, quinoa, and oats. These provide fiber and essential nutrients, supporting digestive health.

Healthy Fats:

Include sources of healthy fats, such as avocados, olive oil, and nuts. These fats contribute to overall nutrition and can help with satiety.

Foods to Limit or Avoid with Sjögren's Syndrome:

Caffeine and Alcohol:

Both caffeine and alcohol can contribute to dehydration, exacerbating dryness symptoms. Limit intake and ensure adequate water consumption.

Sugary Foods and Beverages:

Excessive sugar intake can contribute to inflammation and may negatively impact overall health. Limiting sugary foods and beverages is advisable.

High-Sodium Foods:

Excessive salt can contribute to high blood pressure and may pose risks for individuals with Sjögren's, especially those with kidney involvement. Moderation in salt intake is key.

Artificial Sweeteners:

Some individuals may experience worsened symptoms with artificial sweeteners. Be mindful of their presence in sugar-free products and consider alternatives if needed.

Processed and Fried Foods:

Processed and fried foods may contain unhealthy fats and additives. Opt for whole, minimally processed foods to support overall health.

Spicy Foods:

Spicy foods may exacerbate symptoms for some individuals, especially those with mouth and throat dryness. Monitor personal tolerance levels.

Dairy if Lactose Intolerant:

If lactose intolerant, limit or avoid dairy products to prevent digestive discomfort. Opt for lactose-free alternatives.

Potential Allergens:

Identify and avoid any foods that trigger allergic reactions or sensitivities. Common allergens include gluten, nuts, and shellfish.

It's important to note that individual responses to specific foods can vary, and personalized dietary adjustments may be necessary.

Consulting with a registered dietitian or healthcare professional can provide tailored guidance based on individual needs, preferences, and any existing medical conditions.

Additionally, maintaining a well-balanced diet, staying hydrated, and monitoring how specific foods affect symptoms are essential components of managing Sjögren's syndrome through nutrition.

CHAPTER THREE

Healthy Sjogren's Syndrome Recipes

Breakfast

1. Overnight Chia Seed Pudding

Ingredients:

- 2 tbsp chia seeds
- 1 cup almond milk
- 1 tsp honey
- Fresh berries for topping

Instructions:

- Mix chia seeds and almond milk in a jar.
- Add honey and stir well.
- Refrigerate overnight.
- Top with fresh berries before serving.

Cooking Time: Overnight

2. Greek Yogurt Parfait

Ingredients:

- 1 cup Greek yogurt
- 1/2 cup granola
- 1/4 cup mixed berries
- Drizzle of honey

Instructions:

- Layer Greek yogurt, granola, and berries in a glass.
- Drizzle with honey.
- Repeat layers as desired.

Cooking Time: 5 minutes

3. Quinoa Breakfast Bowl

Ingredients:

- 1/2 cup cooked quinoa
- 1/4 cup sliced almonds
- 1/2 banana, sliced
- 1 tbsp maple syrup

Instructions:

- Combine cooked quinoa, sliced almonds, and banana.
- Drizzle with maple syrup.

Cooking Time: 15 minutes (if quinoa isn't pre-cooked)

4. Smoothie Bowl

Ingredients:

- 1 frozen banana
- 1/2 cup frozen berries
- 1/2 cup almond milk
- Toppings: sliced kiwi, shredded coconut

Instructions:

- Blend banana, berries, and almond milk until smooth.
- Pour into a bowl and top with kiwi and coconut.

Cooking Time: 5 minutes

5. Avocado Toast with Poached Egg

Ingredients:

- 1 slice whole-grain bread
- 1/2 avocado, mashed
- 1 poached egg
- Salt and pepper to taste

Instructions:

- Toast the bread.
- Spread mashed avocado on the toast.
- Top with a poached egg and season with salt and pepper.

Cooking Time: 10 minutes

6. Oatmeal with Almond Butter and Banana

Ingredients:

- 1/2 cup rolled oats
- 1 cup almond milk
- 1 tbsp almond butter
- Sliced banana for topping

Instructions:

- Cook oats with almond milk.
- Stir in almond butter.
- Top with sliced banana.

Cooking Time: 10 minutes

7. Egg White Veggie Omelette

Ingredients:

- 3 egg whites
- 1/4 cup diced bell peppers
- 1/4 cup spinach
- 1 tbsp feta cheese

Instructions:

- Whisk egg whites and pour into a heated pan.
- Add bell peppers and spinach.
- Once set, fold in half and sprinkle with feta.

Cooking Time: 10 minutes

8. Peanut Butter Banana Wrap

Ingredients:

- 1 whole-grain tortilla
- 2 tbsp peanut butter
- 1 banana, sliced

Instructions:

- Spread peanut butter on the tortilla.
- Add sliced banana and roll it up.
- Cooking Time: 5 minutes

9. Cottage Cheese and Pineapple Bowl

Ingredients:

- 1/2 cup cottage cheese
- 1/2 cup fresh pineapple chunks
- 1 tbsp chopped mint

Instructions:

- Combine cottage cheese and pineapple.
- Sprinkle with chopped mint.

Cooking Time: 5 minutes

10. Almond Flour Pancakes

Ingredients:

- 1 cup almond flour
- 2 eggs
- 1/2 cup almond milk
- 1 tsp vanilla extract

Instructions:

- Mix almond flour, eggs, almond milk, and vanilla.
- Cook on a griddle until golden.

Cooking Time: 15 minutes

11. Fruit Salad with Mint

Ingredients:

- Assorted fresh fruits (berries, melon, grapes)
- Fresh mint leaves
- 1 tbsp honey

Instructions:

- Combine fresh fruits.

- Drizzle with honey and garnish with mint.

Cooking Time: 10 minutes

12. Brown Rice Breakfast Bowl

Ingredients:

- 1/2 cup cooked brown rice
- 1/4 cup sliced almonds
- 1/2 cup sliced strawberries
- 1 tbsp honey

Instructions:

- Mix brown rice, almonds, and strawberries.
- Drizzle with honey.

Cooking Time: 15 minutes (if rice isn't pre-cooked)

13. Coconut Chia Seed Pudding

Ingredients:

- 2 tbsp chia seeds
- 1 cup coconut milk
- 1/4 cup shredded coconut
- Sliced mango for topping

Instructions:

- Mix chia seeds and coconut milk in a jar.
- Stir in shredded coconut.
- Refrigerate overnight.
- Top with sliced mango.

Cooking Time: Overnight

14. Turmeric and Ginger Infused Tea

Ingredients:

- 1 cup hot water
- 1/2 tsp turmeric powder
- 1/2 tsp grated ginger
- 1 tsp honey

Instructions:

- Steep turmeric and ginger in hot water.
- Stir in honey.

Cooking Time: 5 minutes

15. Spinach and Mushroom Breakfast Wrap

Ingredients:

- 1 whole-grain tortilla
- 1/2 cup sautéed spinach and mushrooms
- 1 scrambled egg
- Feta cheese (optional)

Instructions:

- Fill the tortilla with sautéed spinach and mushrooms.
- Add scrambled egg and feta if desired.
- Roll it up.

Cooking Time: 15 minutes (including sautéing)

Lunch

1. Quinoa Salad with Roasted Vegetables

Ingredients:

- 1 cup quinoa

- Assorted vegetables (bell peppers, cherry tomatoes, zucchini)
- Olive oil
- Fresh lemon juice
- Salt and pepper to taste

Instructions:

- Cook quinoa according to package instructions.
- Toss vegetables in olive oil, salt, and pepper, then roast until tender.
- Mix cooked quinoa with roasted vegetables.
- Drizzle with fresh lemon juice and serve.

Cooking Time: 30 minutes

2. Salmon and Avocado Wrap

Ingredients:

- Grilled salmon fillet
- Whole-grain wrap
- Sliced avocado
- Greek yogurt sauce (Greek yogurt, lemon juice, dill)
- Lettuce leaves

Instructions:

- Grill salmon until cooked.
- Spread Greek yogurt sauce on the wrap.
- Place salmon, sliced avocado, and lettuce on the wrap.
- Roll tightly and cut in half before serving.

Cooking Time: 20 minutes

3. Lentil and Vegetable Soup

Ingredients:

- 1 cup lentils
- Mixed vegetables (carrots, celery, spinach)
- Vegetable broth
- Garlic, minced
- Cumin, coriander, salt, and pepper to taste

Instructions:

- Rinse lentils and cook in vegetable broth until tender.
- Sauté minced garlic in olive oil, add chopped vegetables, and cook until softened.

- Combine vegetables with lentils and season with cumin, coriander, salt, and pepper.

Cooking Time: 40 minutes

4. Spinach and Chickpea Salad

Ingredients:

- Fresh spinach leaves
- Canned chickpeas, drained
- Cherry tomatoes, halved
- Feta cheese
- Balsamic vinaigrette dressing

Instructions:

- Toss spinach, chickpeas, cherry tomatoes, and feta in a bowl.
- Drizzle with balsamic vinaigrette dressing.
- Mix well and serve.

Cooking Time: 15 minutes (no cooking required)

5. Turkey and Vegetable Stir-Fry

Ingredients:

- Lean ground turkey
- Broccoli florets
- Bell peppers, sliced
- Soy sauce
- Ginger, minced
- Brown rice

Instructions:

- Cook ground turkey in a pan until browned.
- Add sliced vegetables and minced ginger, stir-frying until tender.
- Pour in soy sauce and cook until heated through.
- Serve over cooked brown rice.

Cooking Time: 25 minutes

6. Greek Chicken Salad

Ingredients:

- Grilled chicken breast, sliced
- Romaine lettuce

- Cucumber, diced

- Cherry tomatoes, halved

- Kalamata olives

- Feta cheese

- Olive oil and lemon dressing

Instructions:

- Arrange lettuce on a plate and top with grilled chicken, cucumber, tomatoes, olives, and feta.

- Drizzle with olive oil and lemon dressing.

Cooking Time: 20 minutes

7. Sweet Potato and Chickpea Bowl

Ingredients:

- Roasted sweet potatoes

- Canned chickpeas, drained and roasted

- Quinoa

- Greek yogurt sauce (Greek yogurt, lemon juice, garlic)

- Fresh cilantro, chopped

Instructions:

- Roast sweet potatoes and chickpeas in the oven.
- Cook quinoa according to package instructions.
- Assemble a bowl with quinoa, roasted sweet potatoes, and chickpeas.
- Top with Greek yogurt sauce and fresh cilantro.

Cooking Time: 40 minutes

8. Caprese Wrap

Ingredients:

- Whole-grain wrap
- Sliced turkey or chicken breast
- Fresh mozzarella, sliced
- Tomatoes, sliced
- Basil leaves
- Balsamic glaze

Instructions:

- Layer turkey or chicken, mozzarella, tomatoes, and basil on the wrap.
- Drizzle with balsamic glaze.

- Roll tightly and cut before serving.

Cooking Time: 15 minutes (no cooking required)

9. Shrimp and Quinoa Salad

Ingredients:

- Cooked shrimp
- Quinoa
- Avocado, diced
- Cherry tomatoes, halved
- Cilantro, chopped
- Lime juice
- Salt and pepper to taste

Instructions:

- Combine cooked shrimp, quinoa, diced avocado, tomatoes, and cilantro in a bowl.
- Squeeze lime juice over the salad and season with salt and pepper.

Cooking Time: 25 minutes

10. Mediterranean Hummus Bowl

Ingredients:

- Hummus
- Quinoa or couscous
- Cherry tomatoes, halved
- Cucumber, sliced
- Olives
- Feta cheese
- Olive oil drizzle

Instructions:

- Cook quinoa or couscous according to package instructions.
- Arrange a bowl with a base of hummus, topped with quinoa, tomatoes, cucumber, olives, and feta.
- Drizzle with olive oil before serving.

Cooking Time: 20 minutes

11. Tuna and White Bean Salad

Ingredients:

- Canned tuna, drained

- Cannellini beans, drained and rinsed

- Red onion, finely chopped

- Parsley, chopped

- Olive oil and lemon juice dressing

- Salt and pepper to taste

Instructions:

- Mix tuna, white beans, red onion, and parsley in a bowl.

- Drizzle with olive oil and lemon juice dressing.

- Season with salt and pepper.

Cooking Time: 15 minutes (no cooking required)

12. Veggie and Quinoa Stuffed Bell Peppers

Ingredients:

- Bell peppers, halved

- Quinoa, cooked

- Black beans, drained and rinsed

- Corn kernels

- Salsa

- Cumin, chili powder, salt, and pepper to taste

Instructions:

- Preheat the oven and roast halved bell peppers.
- Mix cooked quinoa, black beans, corn, salsa, and spices in a bowl.
- Stuff bell peppers with the quinoa mixture and bake until peppers are tender.

Cooking Time: 40 minutes

13. Chicken and Vegetable Skewers

Ingredients:

- Chicken breast, cut into cubes
- Bell peppers, cherry tomatoes, and red onion, cut into chunks
- Olive oil
- Garlic, minced
- Lemon juice
- Oregano, salt, and pepper to taste

Instructions:

- Marinate chicken and vegetables in olive oil, minced garlic, lemon juice, and spices.
- Thread onto skewers and grill until chicken is cooked through.
- Serve with a side of quinoa or brown rice.

Cooking Time: 30 minutes

14. Egg Salad Lettuce Wraps

Ingredients:

- Hard-boiled eggs, chopped
- Greek yogurt
- Dijon mustard
- Celery, finely chopped
- Lettuce leaves

Instructions:

- Mix chopped eggs, Greek yogurt, Dijon mustard, and celery in a bowl.
- Spoon the egg salad into lettuce leaves to create wraps.

Cooking Time: 15 minutes (including boiling eggs)

15. Vegetable and Brown Rice Stir-Fry

Ingredients:

- Mixed vegetables (broccoli, carrots, snap peas)
- Tofu or chicken, cubed
- Brown rice, cooked
- Soy sauce
- Ginger, minced
- Garlic, minced
- Sesame oil

Instructions:

- Stir-fry tofu or chicken in sesame oil until browned.
- Add mixed vegetables, minced ginger, and garlic, cooking until tender.
- Pour in soy sauce and cook until heated through.
- Serve over cooked brown rice.

Cooking Time: 25 minutes

Dinner

1. Grilled Salmon with Lemon-Dill Sauce

Ingredients:

- 4 salmon fillets
- 2 tablespoons olive oil
- Salt and pepper to taste
- 2 tablespoons fresh dill, chopped
- Juice of 1 lemon

Instructions:

- Preheat grill to medium-high heat.
- Brush salmon with olive oil and season with salt and pepper.
- Grill salmon for 4-5 minutes per side, or until cooked through.
- In a small bowl, mix lemon juice and chopped dill for the sauce.
- Drizzle the lemon-dill sauce over the grilled salmon before serving.

Cooking Time: 15 minutes

2. Quinoa and Vegetable Stir-Fry

Ingredients:

- 1 cup quinoa, rinsed
- 2 cups mixed vegetables (broccoli, bell peppers, carrots)
- 2 tablespoons soy sauce (low-sodium)
- 1 tablespoon sesame oil
- 2 cloves garlic, minced

Instructions:

- Cook quinoa according to package instructions.
- In a wok or large pan, stir-fry mixed vegetables in sesame oil until tender.
- Add minced garlic and continue cooking for 1-2 minutes.
- Mix in cooked quinoa and soy sauce, stirring until well combined.
- Serve the quinoa and vegetable stir-fry hot.

Cooking Time: 20 minutes

3. Baked Lemon Herb Chicken

Ingredients:

- 4 boneless, skinless chicken breasts
- 2 tablespoons olive oil
- 1 teaspoon dried thyme
- 1 teaspoon dried rosemary
- Zest of 1 lemon
- Salt and pepper to taste

Instructions:

- Preheat oven to 400°F (200°C).
- Rub chicken breasts with olive oil, thyme, rosemary, lemon zest, salt, and pepper.
- Place chicken in a baking dish and bake for 25-30 minutes or until internal temperature reaches 165°F (74°C).
- Let the chicken rest for a few minutes before serving.

Cooking Time: 30 minutes

4. Lentil and Vegetable Soup

Ingredients:

- 1 cup dried green lentils, rinsed

- 4 cups vegetable broth

- 1 onion, diced

- 2 carrots, chopped

- 2 celery stalks, chopped

- 2 cloves garlic, minced

- 1 teaspoon cumin

- Salt and pepper to taste

Instructions:

- In a large pot, sauté onions, carrots, and celery until softened.

- Add garlic and cumin, cooking for an additional minute.

- Pour in vegetable broth and add lentils. Bring to a boil.

- Reduce heat and simmer for 20-25 minutes or until lentils are tender.

- Season with salt and pepper before serving.

Cooking Time: 40 minutes

5. Roasted Vegetable and Quinoa Salad

Ingredients:

- 1 cup quinoa, cooked
- 2 cups mixed roasted vegetables (zucchini, cherry tomatoes, bell peppers)
- 2 tablespoons balsamic vinaigrette
- 1/4 cup feta cheese, crumbled
- Fresh basil leaves for garnish

Instructions:

- Toss cooked quinoa and roasted vegetables in a large bowl.
- Drizzle with balsamic vinaigrette and toss to coat.
- Sprinkle crumbled feta cheese over the salad.
- Garnish with fresh basil leaves before serving.

Cooking Time: 30 minutes

6. Turkey and Vegetable Skewers

Ingredients:

- 1 pound turkey breast, cut into cubes
- 2 bell peppers, cut into chunks
- 1 red onion, cut into wedges
- 2 tablespoons olive oil
- 1 teaspoon smoked paprika
- Salt and pepper to taste

Instructions:

- Preheat grill or oven broiler.
- Thread turkey, bell peppers, and onion onto skewers.
- Mix olive oil, smoked paprika, salt, and pepper in a bowl.
- Brush the skewers with the olive oil mixture.
- Grill or broil for 15-20 minutes, turning occasionally, until turkey is cooked through.

Cooking Time: 20 minutes

7. Spinach and Feta Stuffed Chicken Breast

Ingredients:

- 4 boneless, skinless chicken breasts
- 2 cups fresh spinach
- 1/2 cup feta cheese, crumbled
- 2 cloves garlic, minced
- Salt and pepper to taste
- 1 tablespoon olive oil

Instructions:

- Preheat oven to 375°F (190°C).
- In a pan, sauté spinach and garlic until wilted.
- Slice a pocket into each chicken breast and stuff with sautéed spinach and feta.
- Season chicken with salt and pepper.
- Heat olive oil in an oven-safe skillet and sear chicken on both sides.
- Transfer the skillet to the oven and bake for 20-25 minutes or until chicken is cooked through.

Cooking Time: 30 minutes

8. Chickpea and Vegetable Curry

Ingredients:

- 1 can chickpeas, drained and rinsed
- 1 cup cauliflower florets
- 1 cup diced tomatoes
- 1 onion, chopped
- 2 cloves garlic, minced
- 1 tablespoon curry powder
- 1 cup coconut milk
- Salt and pepper to taste

Instructions:

- In a pot, sauté onions and garlic until softened.
- Add curry powder and cook for 1-2 minutes.
- Add chickpeas, cauliflower, diced tomatoes, and coconut milk.
- Simmer for 15-20 minutes, stirring occasionally.
- Season with salt and pepper before serving over rice or quinoa.

Cooking Time: 30 minutes

9. Shrimp and Vegetable Stir-Fry

Ingredients:

- 1 pound shrimp, peeled and deveined
- 2 cups broccoli florets
- 1 bell pepper, sliced
- 2 carrots, julienned
- 3 tablespoons soy sauce (low-sodium)
- 1 tablespoon honey
- 1 teaspoon ginger, grated
- 2 cloves garlic, minced

Instructions:

- In a bowl, mix soy sauce, honey, ginger, and garlic to create the sauce.
- In a wok or skillet, stir-fry shrimp until pink and cooked through.
- Add broccoli, bell pepper, and carrots, continuing to stir-fry until vegetables are tender.
- Pour the sauce over the shrimp and vegetables, stirring to coat.
- Serve over rice or noodles.

Cooking Time: 20 minutes

10. Mediterranean Chickpea Salad

Ingredients:

- 2 cans chickpeas, drained and rinsed
- 1 cucumber, diced
- 1 cup cherry tomatoes, halved
- 1/2 red onion, finely chopped
- 1/4 cup Kalamata olives, sliced
- 1/4 cup feta cheese, crumbled
- 2 tablespoons olive oil
- Juice of 1 lemon
- Fresh oregano for garnish

Instructions:

- In a large bowl, combine chickpeas, cucumber, cherry tomatoes, red onion, olives, and feta cheese.
- In a small bowl, whisk together olive oil and lemon juice for the dressing.
- Drizzle the dressing over the salad and toss to combine.
- Garnish with fresh oregano before serving.

Cooking Time: 15 minutes

11. Lemon Herb Baked Cod

Ingredients:

- 4 cod fillets
- 2 tablespoons olive oil
- 1 teaspoon dried thyme
- 1 teaspoon dried rosemary
- Zest of 1 lemon
- Salt and pepper to taste

Instructions:

- Preheat oven to 400°F (200°C).
- Place cod fillets in a baking dish.
- Drizzle with olive oil and sprinkle with thyme, rosemary, lemon zest, salt, and pepper.
- Bake for 15-20 minutes or until fish flakes easily with a fork.

Cooking Time: 20 minutes

12. Brown Rice and Black Bean Bowl

Ingredients:

- 2 cups cooked brown rice
- 1 can black beans, drained and rinsed
- 1 cup corn kernels (fresh or frozen)
- 1 avocado, diced
- 1/4 cup cilantro, chopped
- Lime wedges for serving

Instructions:

- In a bowl, mix brown rice, black beans, corn, avocado, and cilantro.
- Toss the ingredients together until well combined.
- Serve in bowls with lime wedges for squeezing over the top.

Cooking Time: 20 minutes

13. Turkey and Vegetable Lettuce Wraps

Ingredients:

- 1 pound ground turkey

- 1 cup mixed vegetables (carrots, bell peppers, water chestnuts), finely chopped
- 2 tablespoons hoisin sauce
- 1 tablespoon soy sauce (low-sodium)
- 1 teaspoon sesame oil
- Butter lettuce leaves for wrapping

Instructions:

- In a skillet, brown ground turkey until cooked through.
- Add chopped vegetables and cook until softened.
- Stir in hoisin sauce, soy sauce, and sesame oil, mixing well.
- Spoon the turkey and vegetable mixture into lettuce leaves for wrapping.

Cooking Time: 20 minutes

14. Eggplant and Tomato Stacks

Ingredients:

- 2 large eggplants, sliced
- 2 large tomatoes, sliced
- 1 cup fresh mozzarella, sliced

- 1/4 cup fresh basil leaves

- 2 tablespoons balsamic glaze

- Salt and pepper to taste

Instructions:

- Preheat oven to 375°F (190°C).

- Place eggplant slices on a baking sheet and sprinkle with salt. Let sit for 15 minutes.

- Rinse the salt from the eggplant and pat dry.

- On each eggplant slice, layer a slice of tomato, mozzarella, and a basil leaf.

- Repeat the layers and bake for 20-25 minutes or until cheese is melted and bubbly.

- Drizzle with balsamic glaze before serving.

Cooking Time: 25 minutes

15. Vegetable and Tofu Coconut Curry

Ingredients:

- 1 block firm tofu, cubed

- 2 cups mixed vegetables (bell peppers, broccoli, carrots)

- 1 can coconut milk

- 2 tablespoons red curry paste

- 1 tablespoon soy sauce (low-sodium)

- 1 tablespoon brown sugar

- Fresh cilantro for garnish

Instructions:

- In a pan, sauté tofu until lightly browned.

- Add mixed vegetables and continue cooking until vegetables are tender.

- In a separate bowl, whisk together coconut milk, red curry paste, soy sauce, and brown sugar.

- Pour the coconut curry mixture over the tofu and vegetables, simmering for 10-15 minutes.

- Garnish with fresh cilantro before serving over rice.

Cooking Time: 30 minutes

Snack

1. Fruit and Yogurt Parfait:

Ingredients:

- Greek yogurt

- Mixed berries (blueberries, strawberries)

- Granola

- Instructions:

- Layer Greek yogurt, mixed berries, and granola in a glass.

- Repeat layers as desired.

- Serve immediately.

2. Avocado and Tomato Rice Cakes:

Ingredients:

- Rice cakes

- Avocado, sliced

- Cherry tomatoes, halved

- Sea salt and black pepper

Instructions:

- Top rice cakes with sliced avocado and cherry tomatoes.

- Sprinkle with sea salt and black pepper.

Enjoy!

3. Hummus and Veggie Sticks:

Ingredients:

- Hummus (store-bought or homemade)
- Carrot sticks, cucumber slices, bell pepper strips

Instructions:

- Dip vegetable sticks into hummus.
- Enjoy this crunchy and hydrating snack.

4. Chia Seed Pudding:

Ingredients:

- Chia seeds
- Almond milk
- Vanilla extract
- Fresh berries

Instructions:

- Mix chia seeds, almond milk, and vanilla extract in a jar.
- Refrigerate for a few hours or overnight.
- Top with fresh berries before serving.

5. Apple Slices with Nut Butter:

Ingredients:

- Apple slices
- Almond or peanut butter

Instructions:

- Spread nut butter on apple slices.
- Arrange on a plate and enjoy this nutritious snack.

6. Quinoa Salad Cups:

Ingredients:

- Cooked quinoa
- Cherry tomatoes, diced cucumber, feta cheese
- Lemon vinaigrette

Instructions:

- Mix quinoa with veggies and feta.
- Drizzle with lemon vinaigrette.
- Serve in small cups.

7. Trail Mix with Dried Fruits:

Ingredients:

- Mixed nuts (almonds, walnuts)
- Dried fruits (apricots, cranberries)
- Dark chocolate chips

Instructions:

- Mix nuts, dried fruits, and chocolate chips.
- Portion into snack-sized bags.

8. Cucumber and Salmon Bites:

Ingredients:

- English cucumber slices
- Smoked salmon
- Cream cheese

Instructions:

- Spread cream cheese on cucumber slices.
- Top with smoked salmon.

9. Cherry Almond Energy Balls:

Ingredients:

- Dates
- Almonds
- Dried cherries

Instructions:

- Blend dates, almonds, and cherries.
- Form into small energy balls.

10. Coconut Yogurt with Mango:

Ingredients:

- Coconut yogurt
- Fresh mango, diced
- Shredded coconut

Instructions:

- Layer coconut yogurt with diced mango.
- Sprinkle with shredded coconut.

11. Rice Paper Spring Rolls:

Ingredients:

- Rice paper sheets
- Shrimp or tofu
- Fresh veggies (carrots, lettuce, mint)

Instructions:

- Soak rice paper sheets in warm water.
- Fill with chosen ingredients and roll.

12. Sweet Potato Toast with Almond Butter:

Ingredients:

- Sweet potato slices
- Almond butter

Instructions:

- Toast sweet potato slices.
- Spread almond butter on top.

13. Greek Yogurt and Berry Popsicles:

Ingredients:

- Greek yogurt
- Mixed berries
- Honey

Instructions:

- Mix yogurt, berries, and honey.
- Pour into popsicle molds and freeze.

14. Caprese Skewers:

Ingredients:

- Cherry tomatoes
- Mozzarella balls
- Fresh basil leaves

Instructions:

- Skewer tomatoes, mozzarella, and basil.
- Drizzle with balsamic glaze.

15. Cottage Cheese and Pineapple Bowls:

Ingredients:

- Cottage cheese
- Fresh pineapple chunks
- Chopped mint (optional)

Instructions:

- Mix cottage cheese with pineapple.
- Garnish with mint if desired.

CONCLUSION

Adopting a well-thought-out diet is a vital component of managing Sjögren's syndrome and enhancing overall quality of life.

The nutritional strategies discussed, focusing on hydration, anti-inflammatory foods, and mindful choices, can help alleviate specific symptoms associated with the condition.

Incorporating omega-3 rich foods, hydrating fruits and vegetables, and soft, moist snacks can provide relief for dryness symptoms, while avoiding excessive caffeine, alcohol, and sugary foods contributes to overall health.

It is crucial to remember that individual responses to foods may vary, and personal preferences, dietary restrictions, and allergies should be taken into account when planning meals.

Consulting with healthcare professionals, including registered dietitians, can offer personalized guidance to create a diet plan tailored to individual needs.

Maintaining a balanced and nourishing diet, coupled with a holistic approach to managing Sjögren's syndrome, contributes to an improved sense of well-being.

By making informed choices, individuals can empower themselves to navigate the challenges of Sjögren's with resilience and focus on optimizing their health.

As always, any significant dietary changes should be made in consultation with healthcare providers to ensure they align with overall health goals and existing medical conditions.

www.ingramcontent.com/pod-product-compliance
Lightning Source LLC
Chambersburg PA
CBHW061006260726

48661CB00005B/2077